taking care of time

Wheelbarrow Books

taking care of time

poems by cortney davis

WHEELBARROW BOOKS • *East Lansing*

Wheelbarrow Books
Michigan State University Press
East Lansing, Michigan 48823-5245

Printed and bound in the United States of America.

27 26 25 24 23 22 21 20 19 18   1 2 3 4 5 6 7 8 9 10

Library of Congress Control Number: 2017944416
ISBN 978-1-61186-274-4 (paperback)
ISBN 978-1-60917-556-6 (PDF)
ISBN 978-1-62895-323-7 (ePub)
ISBN 978-1-62896-323-6 (Kindle)

Book design by Anastasia Wraight
Cover design by Erin Kirk New.
Cover image is "Peony" ©Jonathan Gordon (Jongordon.smugmug.com) and is
used with permission. All rights reserved.

g green Michigan State University Press is a member of the Green Press
press Initiative and is committed to developing and encouraging ecolog-
ically responsible publishing practices. For more information about the Green
Press Initiative and the use of recycled paper in book publishing, please visit
www.greenpressinitiative.org.

Visit Michigan State University Press at *www.msupress.org*

With the publication of Cortney Davis's *Taking Care of Time* the Residential College in the Arts and Humanities Center for Poetry at Michigan State University embarks upon a long-dreamed-of project, the Wheelbarrow Books Poetry Series. Clearly we pay homage to William Carlos Williams and his iconic poem, "The Red Wheelbarrow." Readers will remember the poem begins, "so much depends / upon / [that] red wheelbarrow." We believe that in the early decades of the twenty-first century, a time when technology, politics, and globalization are changing our lives at a pace we could hardly have imagined, so much depends upon our determination to privilege the voices of our poets, new and old, and to make those voices available to a wide audience. So much depends upon providing a retreat, a place of stillness and contemplation, a place of safety and inspiration. So much depends upon our ability to have access to the words of others so that we see— regardless of race, religion, ethnicity, gender, economic situation, or geographic location— that we all share the human condition, that we are more alike than we are different. Poetry helps us do that. Edward Hirsch reminds us that poetry is one solitude speaking to another—across time, across space, across all of our differences. Audre Lorde reminds us that poetry is not a luxury; it is a necessity. Walt Whitman knew that to have great poets, we must create great audiences. We keep all these things in mind as we set out into the world with Wheelbarrow Books. So much depends upon the collaboration of our readers and writers, the intimate ways they will come to know one another.

ANITA SKEEN, WHEELBARROW BOOKS

Rarely do readers have an opportunity to be such close nonpartisan witnesses in the complex realms of illness and recovery—as we do in *Taking Care of Time* by Cortney Davis. This unforgettable collection of poems is an intimate and powerful window into the fragility and strength of human beings. We stand at the bedsides of patients, we tend, we grow exhausted, we are *in the beds*. Davis has a searing ability to create potent scenes and characters within times of tremulous unknowing: Am I dying? Will I get well? Who is taking care of me? I will never forget arriving at the hospital room in which my father had just died only moments before, to be swept into the arms of a nurse I'd never seen before who gripped me so tightly, repeating, "*Honey, Oh honey.*" Later (when I never saw her again either) I wondered, is that her specialty? To comfort the first family members who arrive? Cortney Davis has many specialties. Very few poets could describe encounters with patients in all sorts of disarray or delicate transition as movingly as she does. Davis's skills as a nurse practitioner and her unflinching to-the-bone gifts as a poet mix eloquently to create a manuscript that will grip and compel readers. Her voice is tender, thoughtful, and tough, and her gaze focused, penetrating, and always curious about our shared human forms and conditions. This is a great book, not to be missed. It was an honor to select *Taking Care of Time* for the first Wheelbarrow Books Poetry Prize.

Naomi Shihab Nye

The only people who really know anything about medical science are the nurses, and they never tell; they'd get slapped if they did.

—DJUNA BARNES, *NIGHTWOOD*

Contents

taking care of time

I.

Nursing 101

Silver scissors glistened, the fluted jewel of a nursing pin
nestled against her breast. I was restless,
watching the shirt move over the boy's back

three seats forward. She hushed us, a hiss of cotton against silk,
then she said *pain* and *shot*, and there
in that bright arena, a crescendo of moans like sweet violins.

I learned how cells collide then meld and peel into spheres,
multisided like soccer balls or Rubik's Cubes.
I stabbed oranges until my hands ran with juice, then patients

until my hands rang with grace. I learned the quick save:
airway entered upside down and turned into breath. I learned
to kiss death, my lips seeking those slack mouths, while a boy

waited, flicking his bright cigarette, the burning eye that led me,
my shift over, to his embrace. Even there,
I longed for the corridors where patients slept in silence

thick as grief. Where the night nurse moved
in my favorite dance—
pianissimo, pale through hospital halls.

Selling Kisses at the Diner

It was my second year, my wild year.
I was a student on the evening shift, my boyfriend

would pick me up after work, take me
to an all-night diner where mostly old men lingered—

the homeless, the widowers, the boozers trying to get straight.
We would saunter in past midnight,

me in my proud uniform, white stockings, and Clinic shoes,
him stopping to slap the backs of the guys he knew.

The old men would sing to me, *I'll give you a dollar for a kiss*,
and I'd take their bills, bend to kiss their cheeks

as if I were Florence Nightingale or little sister to the hookers
who loitered outside the diner door. And yet,

pausing here and there to press my lips to those sad lives,
I recognized the power of my first foray into healing.

Mornings We Rolled Pills
into Fluted Cups

Mornings we rolled pills into fluted cups
prim as our caps. We warmed the vial, felt

the resistance of flesh against the needle.
We bathed all those bodies, washed urine from skin

thin as paper, washed young men, all over,
soothed skin that drank up lotion, our hands moved

up the spine, down to buttocks.
We lifted patients, two nurses better than one.

Hands meeting, heads touching, we hoisted
like farmers. Two nurses

make a bed, hands hiding where the sheets tuck.
The sheets are always cool.

Plastic sheets cover the dead—skin
gets mottled in fifteen minutes, cold to touch.

The death stretcher's hard to push,
all covered up, it makes your arms ache.

We held hands with mourners, leaned our bodies
against old men, stood while hands clutched our waists,

pressed our hands on chests, to revive. We laughed
on the way to the morgue, to survive.

Surgical Rotation

He was the first, first death, first cold palm on my heart,
hand of frost, pulse of fear, he was only thirty-five, his wife
waiting in the family area, he was in for a nothing surgery,
bunion of all things, knobby growth not cancer not tumor,
the anesthesiologist gave him the sleepy juice, the patient
went out easy, surgery progressed, skin cut, bone rasp
snips and grinding, nothing, then the gas man gave a little *uh*
and the surgeon looked up, we all looked up, *BP tanking*,
then the storm dam burst, spewed panic like ice
circulating nurse she hit the button and all hell broke, docs
and residents running, me flat against the wall, held breath,
bam bam code cart, sparks and the flash of needles, blood stink,
names of meds in my ears like static, like shiny wires screeching,
then absolute hush, blank eyes, death like a building fell,
death dust rose and settled, everything quiet and gritty,
everyone with their particular duty, nurses here, there
the senior resident given the task, long walk to the waiting room,
speaking the wife's name in his Bombay lilt, her
scream shot all the way back to OR 3 where I stood
struck dumb, enthralled, all of me bright with this
hard desire, *let this be, let this be, let this be my life's work.*

The Nurse's First Autopsy

The senior students said, *don't
look at the face.*

This was a test: weaker girls who
fainted were dismissed. I held my place,
allowed my thoughts to drift

while I observed the race
between two residents who cut
their corpses neatly and with grace.
Organs, scooped out,

sank in stainless bowls. Blood,
once hot, chased
through tortured veins, now stopped.
The doctors drained the heart with ease.
I wondered what

this patient did when living, and yet,
I loved him less
than I was fascinated. Taught well
to separate myself from feeling, I fought

to care *for* but not *about.* Out
came bone from flesh,
the muscles lax, devoid of heat.
I think my eyes burned—then the corpse
was sutured shut.

Apology to the Woman in Room 23

radioactive isotopes inserted into the body may prevent
the recurrence of cancer

The cylinder didn't glow blue,
but we imagined that it might—a death ray
spewing sparks. There were rules.

One nurse in the room for only five minutes,
barely time to say hello
or wash the patient's face,

and we couldn't stand too near her bed
where the invisible ions
beamed a deadly zone we could not cross.

In spite of this, she managed a dreamy look
as we sprinted in like a relay team
offering a piecemeal bath.

Once we had to bribe the aide
to fill the patient's glass with ice. She took
long sips, cold cubes crashing down the tumbler

to her mouth. All the while,
the cancer cells smoldered in her bones,
burning into ash.

In three days she'd grown so weak
the doctors gloved and gowned in aluminum suits
and pulled the spent rod out.

An orderly locked it
in a little vault with six-inch walls
and hauled it off to God-knows-where.

We watched it
roll away. The doctors said we were safe,
but habit dies hard.

We talked fast.
Pain? More juice? The light?
We kept her thick door shut all night.

Stoned

Marion asked for grass. *You know*, she said. *It's true.*
It's not the dying, but the pain.

Her friends brought in an ounce,
and when Marion grew too weak to build her little cigarettes,

I'd assign a nurse to help.
One day, the supervisor stopped outside our patient's door.

Smell that? she asked.
I shook my head.

You must be used to it, she laughed, *the smell of death.*
Then I could smell it too—

behind the pungent smoke, a scent
slightly off, a little edge to it, like old perfume.

We didn't speak.
Around us, cancer-killing poisons dripped slowly into veins;

everyone was turned and turned again, to keep skin
from breaking down where ribs and bones

poked through, and all the patients' wounds were bound.
Here's what I remember: how Marion laughed

as we nurses with our flimsy cures
pushed every chair against her door

to keep death out. And when we couldn't,
how Marion called us. Hungry. Stoned.

Intubating the Corpse

We try to hold them back,
but the residents already heard

how our patient died.
The most bold strip the sheets, seize her chin.

One takes the steel laryngoscope
and pries it in until the light

finds the woman's vocal cords.
There, a resident says, *aim the tube*

between the cords, and another tries,
fails, then tries again until the blade

slides and lodges in. Others wait their turns,
twirling the bells of stethoscopes or drinking Cokes

while we make frantic calls to those in charge,
pull up the sheets and say, *That's quite enough.*

Finally, we tire, lean with crossed arms
against the wall, the curtains drawn

to hide this scene from passersby. Nurses
watch, and speak only with their eyes.

Angel of Mercy

She has seen the artificial eye afloat in a glass
and the wig in the bald lady's room. Undisturbed,

she directs her flashlight beam onto each sleeping face.
Patients twitch or feel a breeze. If they wake, they find an empty
    room,

bland curtains hanging, nurses' voices like a mother's distant
    song.
The Angel is busy checking, tucking.

She wipes her hands on her skirts, enters the room of her
    favorite,
the boy spun like a chrysalis in cocoons of tubes and stainless
    wires.

He drifts to the *blink-tap* of pumps, the syncope of bellows.
He dreams he is face up in a rowboat, her light a single, red sun

wormed through his lids. She bends to kiss his lips,
her lips dry as wool, then she plucks him from his tethers,

hoists him like a sack. He dreams his boat is rocked by waves.
Tubes snap. Blood sprays the ceiling. The monitor goes blind.

Doctors hurry into the room, flail the boy until he is blue and
    marbled

and they are spent. They cover the shell of his face.

Down the hall, limping, out of breath, the Angel runs, her
        favorite
dancing on her back like awkward wings.

Falling Temperature

The temperature is falling,
the first storm this winter due tomorrow
after months of unexpected warmth, but driving home

I think of *temperature* and how
it climbs higher than you'd think, the human tongue
a bed of coals.

Frosty and mechanical,
we wrap patients in sheets of ice to keep
their brains from cooking. Fevers

plunge fast or else creep down
so slowly we can't save the memory,
then patients wake, confused.

Even our words
are hot: *crisis, defervescence, hyperthermia.*
We know the ache

behind their eyes, how they flush
and feel a desert in their veins, believing they might
burn like paper.

Better off dead, a woman told me,
a tumor in her hypothalamus, a funny word
that made me think of hippos

wading in the Amazon.
Her skin grew thick, the tumor igniting every cell
until she simply fried.

Crispy Critters—that's what nurses call
the burned kids, their bodies hot,
their skin so pink and thin

you want to prick them with a needle,
let some steam escape. Instead,
we peel their flesh

and wrap them tight in gauze
until their body heat drops too low
to register. Like tonight,

when, they say, the temperature is sure to fall.
Driving home, I remind myself that they mean weather.
Weather, I say out loud. That's all.

All Night, Lightning Flared Silently

All night, lightning flared silently
then, a minute later,
thunder over Pittsburgh International Airport.

The bedroom window was hard to open, the neighbor's trees
blue, waiting. Finally,
the rain came, pattering.

In the room, my father's harsh breath drawn in
only partially,
the *pssst chunk* of the oxygen machine, cycling.

By late morning, the sun was sharp.
I sat at the edge of the bed
and stroked his face whenever he cried out.

What memories do we take with us when we go from here?
I'd kept the dresser light dim,
and thunder was like old conversations—

then the sound of a faraway flight.
By noon,
the earth was dry. Nothing left

of the rain, of the long, terrible night,
everything damp and naked,
as it was in the beginning.

Heroics

A slight tremor on the monitor
or a waver in the complex signified a restless patient.

Behind drawn curtains, I'd touch the patient's body
silvered by the IV bottle's light. *Are you*

all right? I'd ask, and watch the bedside screen's
silent sweep, searching for PVCs, SVT,

or the rare run of ventricular fib, the snake
at Eden's gate. If the heart's undulating line

went flat, triggering a high-pitched whine
that wouldn't stop, we'd slather the metallic paddles

like two cold palms and snug them tight.
Hit! we'd cry, and *Hit again!* until the heart's muscle

heaved and wobbled on.
Next morning, I'd tape monitor strips

across the chart to show where the patient died,
then where we arrived. We'd listen

to the saved man sing and watch his heart's line burn—
a solar eclipse we'd seen with our bare eyes.

Teaching CPR

First, shake my shoulders, shout *Annie, Annie!*
Are you OK?
This mannequin was named for me, a girl who drowned;
my parents
had my likeness made—blue sweats, white sneakers,
blond latex hair.
If there's no response, tip back my chin, place your cheek
near my lips.
Look for my breast to rise, *listen* for a rush of air, *feel*
moist breeze
against your cheek. If you don't, seal your lips around
my mouth,
fingers pinch my nose. Big breath in and blow. It feels,
in real life,
or should I say, real death, as if the lungs are sponge, breath
is water.
Now, slide two fingers to feel my carotid artery.
No pulse?
Mark a point a few fingerbreadths above the xiphoid tip
that might break off
when you compress, like that TV action shot of nurses
high astride
as stretchers barrel down the hall, although they rarely
get it right.
Arms straight, you pump *one two three four . . .*
It's like dancing—
our bodies light, partners so well rehearsed we glide, one
    deferring

to the other's grace.
If you're lucky, your patients come around, more like
they come *up*,
lungs frothing, eyes watery and stained by what they've seen.
They found me,
I am told, sodden, blue. They took me home and placed me
in the parlor.
Tonight, another class. Citizens, coming down the stairs,
you'll do fine!
Just remember: *Annie, Annie! Are you OK?* Then, your lips
kissing mine.

Women's Clinic

She digs calloused heels
into the stirrups. Under the sheets, her legs
jut up like ghosts.

I aim the focused glow of light
between the patient's knees—
a scar etches her thighs

like a strand of knotted pearls,
a gift from the man
whose child she carries.

Next patient is a skinny girl,
just fourteen,
her mother standing in the corner.

My hand inside finds
the hard rim of the baby
ten weeks along, and the mother,

raving, *This is all I need!*
Big, sudsy bucket of speculums,
I drop in one more.

Now a girl with earrings round as moons,
their nimbus casting
shadows across the small breasts her old man

found inviting once too often.
I grease two gloved fingers, slip over lateral spines,
thrust back to outline her womb.

Outside, other nervous girls are waiting.
They imagine their babies;
they're already inventing their diminutive names.

The Dark Marks

When I go to wash my lab coats,
there they are, dark marks on the collars, crescent moons
that appear no matter how I soap and shower.

We're all stained: doctors
in surgery, residents in their scrubs, nurses
holding the newly born.
Haven't we all said *six weeks*,
when it would only take three days, or
It seems we've gotten it all, when there it was, all along?

No matter the clean hair, the perfumed neck,
the good, good intentions,
these dark marks remind me we are flesh:

mouths and hands and bodies glorious,
even as we harm. Imperfect, even as we heal.

Hooked Up

Drunk, partying, she
and the man just *hooked up*
she tells me, the college student, the nervous
can't-sit-still woman,
dark-haired, laughing, pierced tongue,
pierced navel, colored threads
braided into bracelets around her wrist,
barely making it through finals,
graduating next spring then
maybe a job, but for today,
she says, the problem is fear,
What if I caught something?, this worry
hooked into her and now
she slides down, eager but not eager
for me to do cultures, blood tests,
to tell her *everything is fine.*
Oh how often I've seen this,
this dread twisted in as if there might be
a tangle inside, shiny, metallic,
like wire, and how each time
I have to pull fear out,
strand by strand,
trying not to weep over this
one more woman *hooked up*,
these barbs deep into flesh,
and how they can only be extracted
with moans and cries, each one
ripping through until

there is no more innocence,
only this woman and me,
helpless to do anything
but go on pulling the hooks from her,
stuffing them into the garbage,
telling her how sweet it must have seemed
that night, how strong
she must be now, how resolute.

Alchemy

The sixteen-year-old with dark eyes slouches on the exam table,
says she wants to keep the pregnancy, knows her life will change.

Her mother sits straight in her chair and tells the daughter,
you should terminate. The girl

catches a breath. Does the mother remember what it was like
before the first flutter, before the belly grew?

The mother cries, and we think she might strike her daughter.
The daughter asks, *would you have gotten rid of me?*

Then she becomes lean, slides off the table, becomes a wolf.
She turns her thin nose to look at us.

None of us try to guess what will happen. The mother
does love her daughter; the daughter loves

her unborn child. At night, howling winds will keep them awake.
They'll walk through snow too cold for any living thing.

The waiting room is crowded. Little girls with newborn babies,
flowered headbands wrapped tight around their skulls.

The Circulating Nurse Enters
the Operating Room

Let her not be blinded by the glare of the spotlight
or distracted by the tangle of plastic tubes,

the stink of anesthesia waiting in its multichambered
monolith of sleep. Let her stand beside her patients

and look into their eyes. Let her say, *we will take care of you.*
Let her understand what it is to be overcome by fear.

Let her secure her mask and turn to the counting and opening,
the writing down. Let her watch closely and, if she has to,

tap a surgeon's shoulder, *watch it*, if he seems on the edge
of contamination. Let the cutting and suturing go well.

Let the blood that saturates the gauze be red; let the organs
be glassy and pink; let the sickness be lifted out

and taken away in a stainless steel bowl. Let her patients awake,
mumbling their thanks. Let the stretchers arrive

and the linens be white. Let the patients be lifted
from the thin table, waving *good-bye, good-bye*

as they are taken to recovery, where other nurses wait
with oxygen, with warm blankets, with eager hands.

Waking

There is nothing
and then, everything at once.

The recovery room hums like high-tension wires
or a neon sign blinking
                    Isn't this a miracle,
                    isn't this a miracle?

You have returned from that vast sleep
during which you forgot the doctor's voice.
Count backward, it said, and you obeyed,
as if you had a choice.

You slid into death's false pocket
jingled like change
to haggle the price of a grave—or so it seemed.

Now armies of hummingbirds
buzz your veins. You hear a radio,
the clock's exaggerated tick.
You've been reborn to skin on sheets,
pain's fire doused by needle stick.

The nurse's mother-face wavers before your eyes.
All the rest, white lies.

It Was a Good Year for Dreams

It was a good year for dreams. They came
    like poems and taught me.
    Everyone was there, especially
    my children. Kittens spilled
    into stairwells like buttons,
    and men followed me, shadows
    darting past locked windows—
    the long "I" that knocks,
    knocks at the door. How to
    escape myself was the question.
    How to dream of Kandahar,
    Kosovo, even Turkey where
    a woman came out of the ruins
    in Ephesus, near the library
    where Saint Sophia stands, frozen.
    You could see through the walls,
    and the books were dust. She
    was our guide—bleached hair,
    a taste for American videos.
    She showed me her bruised eye,
    the red mark across her cheek.
    You must get away, I said when we
    kissed goodbye. It was a hot
    day, sweat like blood, my lips
    like the salty slap of a hand,
first on one side of her face, then on the other.

II.

Becoming the Patient

1.

In the hospital, after the operation
when the clear tube that drained my stomach
felt like fire in my throat
and the intravenous pinched my skin
I saw, like a waking-up dream, a nurse leaning over me
her arm so close all I could see were the blond hairs
and the glistening gold of the bracelet at her wrist
and in that second I thanked God for the beauty
of the bracelet and the arm
that offered the scent of soap

and for the silent tending all those nights
when all I could see was the arm, that glittering gold
even in the dark when drains were emptied
and oxygen adjusted, it was that arm and that
delicate strand
that held me to my life

2.

In the hospital, in the haze of could-die
could-get-better
I came to understand gender
not in the way I'd always thought
male and female
the externals and the assumed
but in how it was sometimes the feminine
my body sought
and other times the masculine
how necessary both

the tender gentle sympathy
and other times
the strength and deference
that lifted and held and did not let me fall

3.

In the hospital when the fever would not go down
and fluid seeped from my veins to swell my skin
when lungs filled with water
and infection devoured muscle and blood
when they offered protein in yellow IVs
and blood in bright red bags
when the blood poured in poured out again
and every breath threatened me
when the CT scan whirred and the machines pinged
and not one test came to my defense
when God abandoned me in the second week
and only the dark night sky looked in
when I thought *I could die* I told myself
and told myself that there were others who suffered
and others who were whole

4.

In the hospital every morning the surgical residents
came by at 5 a.m., blazing on the lights
and standing around the foot of my bed
five or six of them, a nightmare of women and men
asking *how do you feel this morning*
not waiting for my reply but rather
descending upon my body
one listening to my heart and another
pushing my belly, lifting the bandages and
shaking the drainage bag, and two others
at my legs, pressing skin to bone to see how much
edema remained, pressing and pressing
until I said *stop*, and no one knew which one

was hurting me, the belly or the legs
and once when I began to retch the chief resident
said, *she'll be fine*, and as he led them away
each one smacked the hand sanitizer device
on the wall to release the purifying gel
rubbed their hands once or twice
and went on to the next patient

5.

In the hospital my husband stayed
he stayed by my side
when I woke from one surgery and then another
he stayed
when they drew my blood and changed my tubes
when I peed or filled the commode with blood
when I cried he stayed
he didn't leave when I retched
and if I walked he walked with me
gathering my IV lines and holding my arm
if I slept he sat in the corner and waited
when I was in pain he stayed
he stayed after visiting hours were over
and he arrived before they began
when God abandoned me
my husband stayed
when nurses changed shifts
or doctors debated what to do next
when tests couldn't be done until midnight
my husband stayed
when I was in the hospital
my husband stayed

6.

In the hospital the third week
the nurses took pity, moved me to the best room
the executive suite with built-in bookcases

a private shower, a DVD player
with stacks of movies, mostly comedies
and a large TV that hovered over the foot of my bed
staring at me
while in its face I watched the sky's reflection
and yet the machines still hissed and pinged
IVs still pinched
the elderly woman in the next room
cried, *help me, help me*, all night long
and the fluid in my lung became a rising tide
when the doctor drew the fluid out
with a long needle of pain
the specimen was overlooked in the lab
the test ruined
and my fancy room didn't comfort me at all
it just lifted its haughty nose in the air

7.

In the hospital I waited all night
for medication to lull or exhaustion to overcome
but pain meds only made my mind hyperaware
of the chatter of janitors on break
the hum of the family waiting room TV
bursts of laughter or voices that wafted by my room
and when a nurse flicked on the lights to check my vitals
hang a new IV or silence an alarm
I quietly offered my arm, my heart, my belly
and when she left
I watched the mute clock on the wall
and like all sleepless patients
I saw the phantom who waits until night
to seize the second hand
holding it back until the hours drag
in a slow and unremitting crawl

8.

In the hospital as soon as you can stand
you must walk, so I walked
tubes clamped and pinned to my robe
my IV stand a silver circle with four poles
each holding its own swaying bag
the yellow was my food, the red my blood
two for antibiotics, I'd push the rolling stand into the hall
surprised each time
by the hospital's vast, bright life
nurses busy at their stations, residents with their laptops
only the cleaning lady a silent presence
who nodded as I crept by, not sure I'd make
the endless loop past the room with the ice machine
the sandwiches, and pudding I could not eat
then down the long stretch where I'd pass other patients
on their daily stroll
and I could guess their illnesses
a man with prostate cancer, his crimson urine bag
the woman with breast cancer, her bald head and IV chemo
a young man, his tubes like mine
we didn't smile or stop to talk, too afraid
too eager to escape each other's sorrows
and lie down with our own

9.

In the hospital I learned
who I really am
in the midst of suffering I saw
my faults, my lack of faith
I kept notes at my bedside
in an almost unreadable hand
how often I have failed to care for others
what do you do when nothing is left
when you are emptied

when my suffering is relieved I feel no joy
is this despair
if I am to die, may I die soon
suffering has exposed me: intolerant
confused, selfish, unloving
there is nothing that cheers me
is suffering prior to death required
am I being punished
what does my suffering teach others
have I not said thank you enough
what does God want of me
have I totally misunderstood

10.

In the hospital after twenty-six days
I was released
it took hours for the order to be entered
for my nurse to come back from the office
where she was, that very morning, let go
part of a general layoff
she told me as she removed my IV
and tried not to weep
what would I do without her
without Sarah, Debbie, Jeanette, Alex, Elsa
Ana, Leslie, and Miguel, who'd survived Iraq
and held me when I couldn't hold myself
without Jessica and Josyane, who wasn't afraid
to get wet when she bathed me as I stood naked
in the bathroom, who changed my sheets
more often than the rules allowed
I didn't know how I would survive at home
until the just-let-go nurse embraced me
and sickness became a place I left

III.

The Ant's Reprieve

Last night I noticed an ant in the shower stall
and decided not to kill it.

By morning, I had forgotten, turned
on the water and stepped in.
A moment later, a scalded black bead
circled the drain.

But I had spared the ant before,
giving it eight, ten more hours—time
for several dreams!

What benevolent, careless eye
watches me, now?

The Nurse's Pockets

When patients are told they are dying
they say something simple:
I've had a good life or *Who will feed my cats?*
It seems harder on the doctor—
he waits outside the door, stalling,
until the patient confronts him.
So, Doc, what's the verdict?

Soon, a nurse comes to bathe the patient.
There is only the sound of water
wrung from the warm washcloth,
the smell of yellow soap,
and the way she spends time praising
the valley of his clavicle, his hollow mouth.

Then, a morning when the patient leaves,
taking his body. The nurse finds nothing
but the bed with its depression,
its map of sheets she strips.
In the drawer, gumdrops. A comb
woven with light hair, and a book
with certain pages marked.

She takes all these into her pockets.
She has trunks in every room of her home,
full of such ordinary things.

A Patient Tells about Her Suffering

—at first, it was a nagging in her throat,
a cough that stirred itself like a drowsy animal.

For days she went to work, dragged herself around,
went home early. But always, the body is inventive:

soon it became an animal enraged.
Muscles on fire, she felt the room

dipping and rising like a country road.
Nights brought on depression,

a certain desperation, a transparency of flesh
that almost seemed a gift,

something she might dedicate.
And so, she said, she offered every ache, each sleepless hour,

and when her illness seemed to worsen,
she listed all the things she'd done or failed to do.

At last, healing came.
Isn't it odd, she asked, how long the nights can seem,

everyone asleep, only the cold outside and your thoughts,
like owls,

sweeping through the woods on the urgent
downstroke of their wings?

Diagnosis HIV

I don't know why I always say
what I think she wants me to say
when she asks if this infection—
these sores, these lesions, this bad prognosis—
is the result of love she made
with the man now her husband
or could it have been another man,
and does this infection prove
that she's bad, something she
has suspected all along,
or maybe it was just bad luck
or could it be, she asks me, punishment
for the way she beat her children
telling them *shut up, shut up,*
and wouldn't it be better, she asks
if she herself was never born,
her own mother on the streets
like a forecast of her life?—
but then she says, *Still,*
I want to live; I've learned my lesson,
and isn't my whole life about to change?
and every time she asks, I say,
Yes, yes. I'm absolutely sure it will.

Follow-Up: Women's Clinic

Alicia sits on the exam table,
        freckles scattered across her nose,
lower lip

pushed out over clear braces.
        She is twelve, with dark brown hair.
I sit at her feet on my rolling stool,

both her nurse and her confessor.
        The young man came into Alicia's house
while her mother was working.

We don't know and Alicia won't say:
        Did he cajole? Did he
cover her face?

Alicia shivers
        beneath the paper drape and stares
at the beige clinic wall.

In the emergency room
        they opened her legs in the light's glare,
scraped under her nails, swabbed

her throat, raked a tiny comb
        through her pubic hair.
They drew blood,

and sent her home.
     "How can I help you," I ask.
"I'd rather he killed me than raped me,"

is what Alicia replies.
     I reach up, enfold her hands.
I too had to learn that my body was mine.

I help her down,
     give back her skirt, her white cotton *camisa*.
Outside the closed exam room door

Alicia's mother and I wait,
     two women standing guard
while Alicia dresses.

Astronomy

We're waiting for the teacher, me and the other students. In front of us, the room is open to the night. The stars reel in the darkness, *mirabile dictu*, and I sit watching until my friend Loretta comes in and sits with me, cross-legged. We begin to chat just as the teacher arrives. Obviously this is the moment when we should be quiet, but Loretta and I go on gabbing about a nurse we know, how she just had a breast removed for cancer. The nurse is only in her early forties, so Loretta and I *tsk tsk* about how awful this is. For relief, we change the subject and start laughing. I try not to laugh out loud and annoy the teacher, but soon I'm laughing so hard my shoulders shake, my whole body shakes. The class gets involved. They shake when I shake. They laugh when I laugh. Loretta leans over and whispers to me, right in the middle of this, that maybe God doesn't control who gets what after all. Maybe He just throws a handful of ills down on the earth. "He couldn't possible *plan* for someone to get breast cancer," she says. This, of course, is the night before she has her mammogram. Before the biopsy. Before the dime of flesh, the stellar scar.

I'm Afraid of the Brief Empty Space

I'm afraid of the waiting room where patients wear slacks and
    slip-off shoes
and families read last month's magazines;

of the aide who calls my name, staccato and without love,
who walks before me down the long hall, never looking back.

I'm afraid of the johnny coat—its cold exposure—and of the
    black tubing
looped on the wall and the clear tubing hooked to the oxygen
    tank;

of the nurse who comes with her IV bag and hollow needle,
asking my name and why I'm here, as if she doesn't know.

I'm afraid of the orderly who arrives with a wheelchair to roll me
    away,
of the white room and the scrub tech busy with her Mayo tray of
    shiny tools;

of the doctor who waves to me from the scrub room, his mouth
moving under his mask, and of the circulating nurse whose eyes
    say nothing.

I'm afraid of the brief empty space, the metal taste, the ringing
    in my ears,

and the utter blackness into which I fall and do not know I'm
    falling.

I'm afraid of waking in the tilting room, of the circle of curtains
and the microphone voice of the nurse who calls my name;

of her snack of ginger ale and crackers—one fizzes too loudly,
the other breaks with the sound of bone and scatters over my
    body.

I'm afraid of the long wait for pathology, for the prognosis, and
    how
at home when the doctor phones, he asks first how I feel, then if
    I'm alone—

Visiting the Lightning Struck

Imagine Moses, his tablets burned by God,
but this is nature's wrath—a man
whose skin is charred with ragged wounds
where bolts raged, piercing heart and lung.

No holy, dead-aimed stroke,
this summer lightning flash fired his corneas
to opaque glass and burst
his eardrums as if they were balloons.

Did fear come with, before, or after?
And did he see, or simply feel, bones smoke,
eyelids fuse? When his heart stopped,
did he gasp and wait until the tick resumed,

or did the lungs freeze first, then
the other organs fail? How will he think
of picnics after this, how love
August's hazy light, where bees drone air

thick as saturated gauze—until clouds
swell, random ions shift and currents
surge to kiss the ground? They say
he throws off blankets, wants all curtains

drawn. I smell his burns across the hall.
I say his name. I knock upon his door.

Distracted by Blackberries

I am distracted by blackberries, how suddenly I see them
in the bowl on the counter, black and shiny,
their little lobules like so many ants, a gang of them,
oddly quiet, at the same time, quite alive, plump and taut,
as if touching the skin of a blackberry might rupture it,
the juices escaping. And don't they seem a bit ominous?—
how dark, how still, how like a small, burnt organ,
perhaps a brain pried from some charred body,
the *sulcus centralis* still precisely delineated, as if flames
only singed but did not destroy. I am distracted by blackberries
at the approach of autumn, its various anniversaries
of death. So I hold this little not-burnt, not-ant thing,
this glossy frightening blackberry, and decide not to eat it,
not to ingest all the smoke and fire of memory.

On Call: Splenectomy

At 3 a.m., the phone rang.
Car crash, the OR supervisor said,
one fool on a bender.

The guy was singing even
under anesthesia, every breath
volatile as the gas piped

into his lungs. We tipped
the table almost upside down
to keep the rancid ooze

inside his stomach and not
all over us. Skin incision,
then fat and fascia, then

a belly-full of blood
welled up and we bailed
with basins, then our hands.

The guy's spleen was ripped
in half, his gut sprang out
like a pink snake from a can.

I handed clamps and every
stitch I had and the spotlight
burned down on us like fire.

It took hours to sort vessel
from nerve, to fit the knobby
liver below the ribs again.

I've taken pity on you,
left out the really awful part.
But you should see how quiet I am,

cinched in the passenger's seat;
how carefully I slice bread
into my bare hands;

how I curl on my left side to sleep.
And these stories—
how I tame them on the page.

Spring, Summer, Fall and Winter

Spring

Thirty weeks,
and the baby's not moving.

I listen to deep silence.

Then, the belly wakes.
From beneath the mountain
thunder singing.

Summer

The final day of OB rotation
the medical student has a choice—
see the last patient of the day
or run to the coffee shop for a milkshake.

Milkshake wins!

What will I say when they ask me
was he dedicated?

Fall

Why did you do this? Why did you order that?

Full of indignation, the chief resident
attacks me

like the attending doctors
attacked her this morning.

Winter

There, on my patient's cervix, a red spot
like a berry.

Today, I see her again,
shuffling her way to the bathroom
without her uterus, without her cancer.

She looks so much smaller.

The Vocation of Illness

Today, when he speaks about holiness, the priest says
that some people have the vocation of illness. I think about this

all the way home, the gray-spired church growing smaller
in my rearview mirror, and the vocation of illness looming

before me like a re-run movie, like when I was a new nurse
at St. Joseph's and my first patient was a woman

dying of a brain tumor, before all the sweet nectars of relief
we have today, before the precise knife and bitter healing
      poisons.

I stood beside her bed as she writhed and groaned,
the harsh white sheets tossed and tugged into disarray.

As I straightened them, as I offered water, company, a back rub,
I'd listen to her constant moan, a long low sound

that rose into a shriek and then receded, like a fierce surf
that roiled and thundered in, then hissed back into the endless,

deepest, darkest blue. When I worked the night shift, I'd find her
still awake, eyes wide, voice hoarse from constant keening.

And today, after all this time, I learn that she was holy,

immolated on a cross I couldn't see. *Hello, woman who died in
agony.*

Can you hear me? Have your cries turned to singing?
Do you stand before the face of God?

There Are No Poems at Hospital Management Meetings

The CEO has a wary gaze; the executive women
wear pearls. We nurses
settle into the audience while poems hide

on other floors—in rooms where we measure cost
in milligrams of morphine, liters of blood;
where *how many more treatments?*

or *how many more days?*
are the only questions on the agenda.
What does this say about management meetings, or poems?

That there are different ways of thinking
about the same thing? Black and white *vs.* metaphor—
or sometimes you save and sometimes you spend?

Today, management talks about fiscal responsibility,
how to cut costs to yield better growth. I
mishear, think they said *bitter* but hold my tongue.

The poems recoil, a slithering sound.
All day, patients polish their diamonds of pain.
Soon, we will pry the dimes from their eyes.

Killing the Nurse in the House

Whenever I felt the shadow of her wing or the radiance of her halo upon my page, I took up the inkpot and flung it at her. She died hard.
—Virginia Woolf

In all those old reruns, she has hair that fits perfectly under that little white pancake hat. She stands up when the doctor arrives, hands him the chart, smiles, and recites the lab work perfectly: *Sodium 145, Potassium 3.2.* While the doctor strips back the patient's sheet and pokes him in the belly, the nurse pours fresh water into the patient's bedside glass and throws away the bloodied gauze. Then she walks with the doctor out to the desk, waits with her pen poised. The doctor notices her body, intriguing under the white, stainless shield of her uniform. She notices him noticing and poses, hip at an angle. He imagines her following him to the ends of the earth dressed in a white teddy and thigh-high hose. He speaks, giving his orders, and she records every word: *Run the IV at 100 cc per hour. Give Ampicillin 500 mgm STAT.* This nurse, the one every patient wants, leaning on their call bells for her attention, thinks she has the answer to pain, incontinence, bleeding, *and* death. This is her—young! This is her—brilliant! This is her—luscious and mute! Kill her! Kill her! That's all you can do.

I Want To Work in a Hospital

where it's okay
to climb into bed with patients
and hold them—
pre-op, before they lose
their legs or breasts, or after,
to tell them
they are still whole.

Or postpartum,
when they have just returned
from that strange garden,
or when they are dying,
as if somehow because I stay
they are free to go.

I want the daylight
I walk out into
to become the flashlight they carry,
waving it
as we go together
into their long night.

My Evidence

When I saw dust settling,
the road black and gritty,

and noticed the air
shimmering as it lowered closer to the earth

like a soft blanket suffocating
the damp September

mornings that had morphed seamlessly
into November's

crowded table
of berries, sweets, and yellow corn,

just before the hospital phoned
to say Mother had called my name,

familiar syllables
caught in her throat,

I'd already detected her leaving
in my own body

and so while she paused
at the end of her journey,

which was also the beginning,
I rushed to her,

hurrying
as I'd never hurried before.

Twelve Thousand Years Ago

Twelve thousand years ago, Sanibel Island rose from the sea,
a coral reef hidden, then revealed.

Having breakfast on a rented verandah, I watch the pale blue
    Gulf of Mexico
disappear into the pale blue sky

and the mother who walks her three-year-old toward the sand.
When he complains

about the rough path, she lifts him to her hip.
In Pittsburgh, when my father was dying, I dripped morphine
    under his tongue

every hour, every half hour,
every twenty minutes. *Don't be afraid*, the hospice nurse told me,

to give whatever will carry him.

Hospice

At dusk, Father takes me for a ride in his maroon Buick LaSalle. As we drive along, I notice Mother standing in an empty lot, dressed in a Jackie Kennedy suit and pillbox hat. I shout to my dad, *Stop! Stop!* I'm shocked to see her—more than that, elated, as if we've been given a second chance. I open the car door and rush out, waving. She runs to me with childlike abandon, arms outstretched. Then I realize she doesn't know me. She's just as confused as she was the month before she died. I help Mother into the back seat and buckle her in. No one speaks. My father drives, dazed, staring ahead as the car drifts and wanders. He seems overwhelmed, his eyes glazed and watery, as if he can't possibly go through this again. He stops the car. A policeman approaches, flipping open his ticket book. *It's alright*, I say, patting my father's arm. *It'll be over soon.*

Taking Care of Time

Yesterday it was a thousand small coins
ringing in your pocket—your hand dipped in, scooping three
at a time, giving them away. Sometimes, you'd drop one
in the lush grass, unaware it was lost.

Today time comes in a different disguise:
a bolt of fine silk, vermillion or blue, you measure it
carefully, like a woman preparing to sew.

Tomorrow, *watch out*, it comes as thunderstorm,
slant rain, February blizzard that drives you inside.
Insomniac, you pace
and curse the glow of computer screen, television, radio.

Soon enough, time may be difficult to recognize.
You might mistake it
for an elderly coughing man or a woman overrun with grief.
Do not stop your ears against its cry:

return any small change;
cherish every moment under the leaden sky.

Finding What You Didn't Expect

It might be something as bland as a handkerchief
wadded deep in a pocket,
or something luckier, the five-dollar bill you thought you'd lost
or spent foolishly on the china horse with the nicked ear,
but oh, how you loved the fragile roses
and the green stems someone painted by hand.
Can you see her,
the girl in a factory in Taiwan, her elbow braced on the table,
paint pots around her like little jewels, the green stem
flowing from the brush's tip?—and all the while she's
    remembering
how she once saw the stained glass windows of Sainte-Chapelle,
how last night she danced in a borrowed pair of alligator heels,
humming "Eleanor Rigby" and plotting her own escape.

Maybe it's a ticket stub from a movie you saw last year
but now can't recall, only the final scene, a fiery car crash,
the way the closing credits rolled over the ambulance wail, the
    men running
as you walked out
blinking into the light. If you're lucky, you might find
the one true answer to the one great question you've carried
    with you
since fifth grade, one that begins either *Why?* or *When?* and now
    you wonder
why you've never searched for it before.

In Taiwan, the girl rinses her brush, licks the bristles
into a perfect eyelash, shuts her paint pots inside a wooden box,
and ties a scarf around her hair because it's begun to rain,
like it might have when Eleanor Rigby
picked up the rice in a church where a wedding had been, the girl
    waiting
for the melody, the right words,
as she walks past red brick shops toward Qingshui Temple,
not expecting anything, not an old ticket stub in her pocket
or even a miracle, and just then,

four thousand miles away,
you're driving I-95 into New York City, recalling, out of nowhere
that August you were eighteen, longing to disappear,
wind blowing your hair, white blouse billowing, mind spinning
    you
into another life,
when suddenly you swerve to miss a car or a deer leaps out,
and all you can do is cry, *Oh God, oh God,*
that's how close you've come to the final scene, the bent metal,
steam hissing from the radiators, medics running,
the credits rolling,
        best boy, musical direction, editing,
after which everyone stands up,
the girl in Taiwan crosses the street, and you,
you've pulled off the highway, the moon in Venus, the sun in
    Sagittarius
and *that's* when you see it—
        a golden horse, like a statue, grazing in a field of yellow
          roses,
and on your watch's face the second hand clicks forward, *next,*
    next second, next.

First Night at the Cheap Hotel

Tonight, the moon is almost full, its glow filtered
through my window's small, square screen.
Down the hall, a man coughs and coughs.
There are women's voices too, tinny, high,
like a sound from childhood,
the fluted, aluminum milk bottle caps
Mother once pierced and jangled on a string.
In my room, the middle note of the air conditioner
and something caught inside the fan, rattling—no, crackling—
like the crackling of air under skin, *crepitus*.

Being here is like being sick in a hospital ward
without the lovely, muffling glove of illness.
In hospital, I would be drowsy, drugged into a calm
that accepts the metal door's clang,
the heavy footfall right outside my door.
All these, proof of life,
and there would be a nurse too, holding my wrist,
counting and nodding, only a silhouette in the dark.

She'd stand beside me, as my mother did,
holding her fingers to her lips, saying *shhh, shhh*,
and, like a child,
feverish, safe,
I would close my eyes and sleep.

The Snake Charmer

I dream that I am a nurse, and she is a woman in a turban. Both of us sit at the roadside. Her snakes crawl all over me. Cobras and baby rattlers and green slugs and earthworms with cinched waists tickle my arms, my hands, my thighs. The snake charmer is impressed that I'm not afraid. Other people step around us, oblivious to the danger. Are they blind? But the woman senses that I am like her. "Do you know the black mamba?" she asks.

Yes. Yes, I do.

Author's Acknowledgments

My gratitude to the editors of the journals in which these poems, some in earlier versions, first appeared.

Alimentum: The Literature of Food: "Selling Kisses at the Diner," "Distracted by Blackberries"

American Journal of Nursing: "Heroics," *American Journal of Nursing* 100, no. 1 (January 2000) and "A Patient Tells about Her Suffering," *American Journal of Nursing* 113, no. 12 (December 2013). Reprinted with permission.

American Nurse Today: "On Call: Splenectomy" [originally published as "Splenectomy"], *American Nurse Today*, October 2006, *AmericanNurseToday.com*. Copyright © 2017 Health-Com Media. All rights reserved.

Annals of Internal Medicine: "Teaching CPR," "Twelve Thousand Years Ago"

Antigonish Review: "Astronomy"

Ars Medica: "Apology to the Woman in Room 23"

Bellevue Literary Review: "I Want To Work in a Hospital," "I'm Afraid of the Brief Empty Space"

Caduceus: "Women's Clinic" [originally published as "Bridgeport Clinic"]

Conclave: A Journal of Character: "Hospice"

Descant: "Finding What You Didn't Expect"

Journal of the American Medical Association: "Visiting the Lightning Struck," *The Journal of the American Medical Association* 265, no. 11, p. 1384, and "Waking," *The Journal of the*

American Medical Association 269, no. 22, p. 2819. Copyright © 1991, 1993 American Medical Association. All rights reserved. Reproduced with permission from *The Journal of the American Medical Association.*

Journal of Medical Humanities: "Falling Temperature," "Intubating the Corpse," *Journal of Medical Humanities* 17, no. 4 (1996). Republished with permission from the *Journal of Medical Humanities.*

Labor: Studies in Working-Class History of the Americas: "The Nurse's First Autopsy"

Lancet: "Mornings We Rolled Pills into Fluted Cups" [originally published as "Touch"], *The Lancet* 350 (1997). Reprinted with permission from Elsevier.

Literature and Medicine: "Angel of Mercy" [originally published as "Nurse as Angel of Mercy"], *Literature and Medicine* 11, no. 1 (1992): 88–89. Copyright © 1992 The Johns Hopkins University Press. Reprinted with permission from Johns Hopkins University Press.

Mission at Tenth: "Follow-Up: Women's Clinic"

Ms. Magazine: "It Was a Good Year for Dreams" Copyright © 2004. Reprinted with permission from *Ms. Magazine.*

MSM: Mens Sana Monographs: "Taking Care of Time"

PULSE: Voices from the Heart of Medicine: "My Evidence," "The Circulating Nurse Enters the Operating Room," "Spring, Summer, Fall and Winter"

Rattle: "Diagnosis HIV"

Reflections on Nursing: "Nursing 101" [originally published as "Career Day"]

Sentence: A Journal of Prose Poetics: "Killing the Nurse in the House"

Sun: "The Ant's Reprieve"

The Healing Muse: A Journal of Literary and Visual Arts: "Becoming the Patient" [originally published as "In the Hospital"]

Underground Voices: "Hooked Up," "First Night at the Cheap Hotel"

Workers Write! Tales from the Clinic: "There Are No Poems at Hospital Management Meetings," "The Dark Marks"

"The Nurse's Pockets" first appeared in *Between the Heartbeats: Poetry and Prose by Nurses*, edited by Cortney Davis and Judy Schaefer (Iowa City: University of Iowa Press, 1995).

"Stoned" first appeared in *Poetry in Medicine: An Anthology of Poems about Doctors, Patients Illness and Healing*, edited by Michael Salcman (New York: Persea, 2015).

I offer my deepest gratitude to Naomi Shihab Nye, Anita Skeen and Laurie Hollinger of the Center for Poetry at Michigan State University; to Julie Loehr, Elise Jajuga, Kristine Blakeslee, Julie Reaume, Annette Tanner, and all those in front of and behind the scenes at Michigan State University Press who midwifed this book gently into the world. I am indebted to L. N. Allen, Meg Lindsay, Charlotte Friedman, Jean Sands, Judson Scruton, Sondra Zeidenstein, and my husband, Jon Gordon. Their wise counsel and support have been invaluable.

As always, this collection is dedicated to my family.

Series Acknowledgments

We at Wheelbarrow Books have many people to thank without whom *Taking Care of Time* would never be in your hands. We begin by thanking all those writers who submitted manuscripts to the first Wheelbarrow Books Poetry Prize. We want to single out the finalists—Carol Barrett, Ruth Moon Kempher, Donald Levering, and Robert Miltner—whose manuscripts moved and delighted us and which we passed onto the judge, along with Cortney Davis's, for her final selection. We thank that judge, Naomi Shihab Nye, for her thoughtful selection of the winner and her critical comments offered earlier in this book.

Our thanks go to Grace Carras, Erin Lammers, Sydney Meadowcroft, Cindy Hunter Morgan, Alexis Stark, Sarah Teppen, and Arzelia Williams for their careful reading of manuscripts and insightful commentaries on their selections, and especially to Laurie Hollinger, assistant director at the Residential College in the Arts and Humanities Center for Poetry, who also read all the manuscripts and provided the logistical aid and financial wizardry for this project. Sarah Teppen designed our Wheelbarrow Books logo, which makes us smile every time we see it.

We also thank Stephen Esquith, dean of the Residential College in the Arts and Humanities, who has given his continued support to the Center for Poetry and Wheelbarrow Books since their inceptions. As we began thinking seriously about Wheelbarrow Books, conversation with June Youatt, provost at Michigan State University, was encouraging, and MSU Press director Gabriel Dotto and assistant director and editor in chief Julie Loehr were eager to support the efforts of poets to continue to reach an eager audience. We cannot thank you enough for having the faith in us, and the love of literature, to collaborate on this project.

Thanks to our current editorial board—Sarah Bagby, Mark Doty, Carolyn Forché, George Ellenbogen, Thomas Lynch, and Naomi Shihab Nye—for believing Wheelbarrow Books was a worthy undertaking and lending their support and their time to our success.

Finally, to our patrons: without your belief in the Wheelbarrow Books Poetry Series and your generous financial backing we would still be sitting around the conference table adding up our loose change. You are making it possible for poets who have never had a book of poetry published, something becoming harder and harder these days with so many presses discontinuing their publishing of poetry, to find an outlet for their work as well as supporting the efforts of established poets to continue to reach a large and grateful audience. We name you here with great admiration and appreciation: Beth Alexander, Mary Hayden, Jean Krueger, Patricia and Robert Miller, and Brian Teppen.